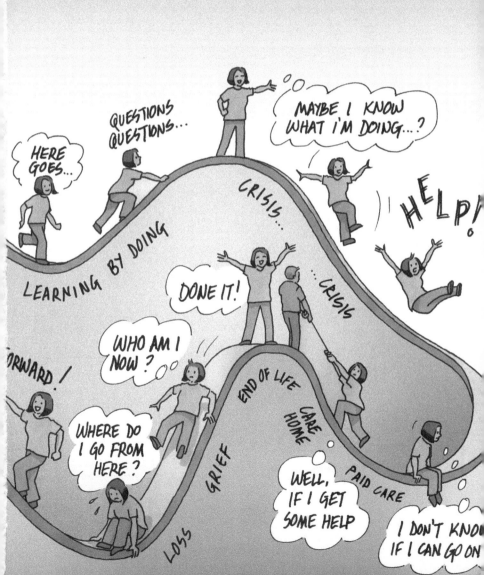

THE ROLLERCOASTER OF

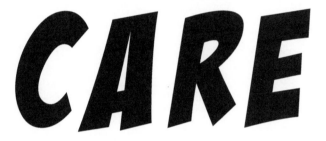

*How to Deal with the Emotional Experience
of Caring for Older People*

THERESA POLLARD and

JENNIFER SAYER

Matador
9 Priory Business Park,
Wistow Road, Kibworth Beauchamp,
Leicestershire. LE8 0RX
Tel: 0116 279 2299
Email: books@troubador.co.uk
Web: www.troubador.co.uk/matador
Twitter: @matadorbooks

ISBN 978 1838591 113

British Library Cataloguing in Publication Data.
A catalogue record for this book is available from the British Library.

Printed and bound by CPI Group (UK) Ltd, Croydon, CR0 4YY
Typeset in 11pt Adobe Garamond Pro by Troubador Publishing Ltd, Leicester, UK

Matador is an imprint of Troubador Publishing Ltd

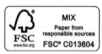

To Jenny's mum and Theresa's Auntie Marie,
without whom this book would never have been written.

Contents

Acknowledgements

We have had many ups and downs as we have completed this book! The journey has had many challenges, and we have much to reflect on, and many people to be grateful for.

In particular we want to thank Mark, Theresa's husband, for his support, patience and practical help throughout the process.

We much appreciate those who have listened to ideas, taken time to read and make suggestions, and given us encouragement when we most needed it. Thanks to Mike, Jenny's brother, who gave us a Canadian perspective and caused us to rewrite the first two chapters, to Dawn who addressed continuity and stimulated the cartoon drawing! Thanks to Mike, Christine and John for commenting on relevance and readability.

Thanks to friends and family, too many to mention, who have used their own uniqueness to keep us going whether by sharing their own experience of caring, prayer, or taking us out for time out! We appreciate you all!

Most important are the people who agreed to being interviewed about their experience of caring. This was not necessarily an easy process because of the feelings (past and present) which were raised up. It was you who kept us going when we might have given up. Thank you for your generosity and honesty in sharing.

Thanks also go to all the people who shared their experience informally with us, keen to ensure that others had the support they had lacked. We again valued your generosity and honesty.

The Contributors

From the start, we wanted examples from experiences other than our own. We did not try to cover every sector of society but used our own networks. All the contributors came from the North-West of England. They had cared for parents, partners, other older relatives or friends, and their ages ranged from forty to eighty. A total of thirty-four different people have been quoted, eight of whom were men. They were a mix of single, partnered, divorced. Some not only had children, but grandchildren.

About the Authors

Theresa comes to this subject with a lot of personal experience of caring and wishes to share her knowledge and to support other carers of older people. She has been a qualified social worker for over thirty years. She has also been involved in social work education linking with many relevant organisations.

Jenny was a long-term carer for her mother and has been very involved in the support of several older friends and their families. She brings a wide knowledge of caring and of relevant organisations from her youth and community work, as a university tutor in social work, and in her current voluntary work for a Christian organisation.

Prologue

Hold on to your hats, we are going on a journey. As a carer for an older person you will recognise many of the paths along the way. Although we appear to be on the same excursion, the experience of caring is unique to each individual. There are many physical and practical demands, but it is the way in which the role challenges your emotions which can be draining and sometimes even damaging.

We have both worked in the social, community and voluntary sectors. We struggled physically and emotionally, however, when it came to caring for an older person close to us. We have written this book from the heart because of our direct experience as carers.

Our intention is to offer support to fellow carers of an older person from our experience, and from the stories of the wonderful variety of carers who contributed to this book. We want to show you that you are not alone in the many ways you are challenged emotionally, and that there is help available. Finally, we want to enable you as a reader to learn from others' experience. We want to help you to recognise the positives that caring can bring to your life, and to develop ways of dealing with the challenges.

Introduction

'Even simple tasks like delivering the shopping left me emotionally drained because I felt guilty having to leave her when she wanted to chat and obviously needed support and company.'
- Trish -

There is much present-day talk about pressures on resources and the difficulties presented by an ageing population. It is on the life of ordinary people, however, that the demands of caring take their toll. This book explores the normal process of ageing and what happens when someone takes on the caring task. It addresses the issues of emotion, identity and evolving relationships as they affect you as a carer. These issues have significant impact on:

- the quality of life of all those involved
- the capacity of the carer to keep going
- the carer's ability to emerge healthily when caring is over.

The book is structured in order to:

1. explore the context which carers need to understand in order to gain outside help
2. encourage and support those of you who are facing the need to take on the role of carer, current carers and those recently bereaved, in relation to elderly relatives
3. identify ways of working together to create a better climate for care.

Our purpose and definition of the role of a carer is:

'Someone without whose help an older person would not be able to cope with practical, emotional, social, physical and spiritual aspects of everyday life.'

This definition is deliberately broad, because our changing society means that not all children are able or prepared to take on the care of their parents. The current more flexible definition and structure of family mean that friends and neighbours are increasingly called into the caring role.

'Care' involves far more than basic tasks like shopping, personal care and hygiene. These tasks are the start of a process in which mutual trust between you as a carer and the person being cared for can be developed. This forms the basis for the emotional and psychological support that becomes necessary as someone's lifestyle becomes more restricted and their needs expand.

Thus the importance of underlying emotions needs to be recognised from the outset. We have both had experience of caring for older people and have learnt the hard way about the cost of acting as an advocate, encourager and provider of emotional support. These make particular demands on your mind, body and spirit, and are often not fully recognised as fundamental to the role of caring. Our intention is to explore ideas and approaches that will enable you as a carer to develop coping strategies and your emotional resilience.

However, the experience of caring is frequently not straightforward. It feels much more like a rollercoaster ride with significant ups and downs, each of which requires different handling:

- The entry into caring is often not clear cut and is quite lengthy.
- Much of the ride is the main caring phase at home when everything is subsumed under the need to survive, whilst keeping the show on the road.
- For some, an additional part of the ride is learning to adjust when the older person needs to go into a residential home.
- A descent ends with bereavement, which entails dealing with loss, and practical and financial issues.

The final stage is what we have termed 'moving on'. When the grief and loss has been gone through, practical issues are sorted, everyone has gone back to their normal lives, what happens to you as the carer then? There is a great deal of work to be done to recover and move on healthily, and carers are often left alone to work this out.

We have interviewed carers from a variety of walks of life, and hope that sharing some of these experiences will help you to recognise that you are not alone in the range of emotions that you may feel, and you will also be able to identify your own unique contribution. You may also identify the special benefits of walking through the last stages of life with someone close to you. It should also help the wider network of people around to understand how to help and support both you as the carer and the person you are caring for.

We have written this book so that you can pick it up and read a section as and when you need to, but can also read the whole thing to get a feel for that ride on the rollercoaster of care, and to know that you are not alone at any time. There is a resource list at the end to help you to follow up specific issues.

RECOGNISING THE SCALE OF THE RIDE

·········

Forewarned is forearmed!

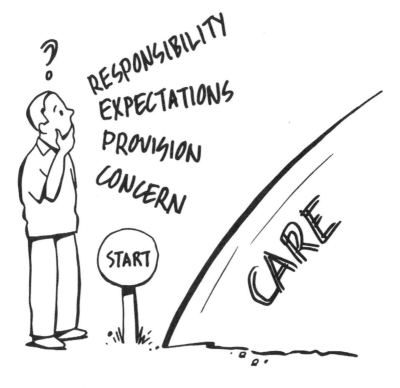

'There are pieces everywhere, no overall picture and therefore the carer can't track services.'

- Sarah -

Before getting on a rollercoaster, we tend to stand back and look at the bigger scale of the ride because the prospect is a bit scary. The same applies when you are contemplating the rollercoaster of care for older people. You need to know what questions to ask, otherwise a great deal of confusion and unnecessary stress can occur.

> *'If I had understood from the very beginning how care services worked and how they saw care, I would have done things very differently and avoided a lot of stress.'*
> **- Mary -**

So, it may help you to ask these three questions:

- How does the world around us understand care?
- Whose responsibility is it?
- Where do I fit in as a carer?

These questions become an essential part of life when you become a carer. You find yourself having to negotiate with organisations which define care by the services they provide, whilst for you it is a very personal experience. Firstly, look at how care has been defined.

The definition of 'care', the noun, is:

> *'The provision of what is necessary for the health, welfare, maintenance and protection of someone or something.'*
> (https://oxforddictionaries.com>care)

However, if you look at the verb 'to care' it is defined as:

'To feel concern or interest, attach importance to something, look after and provide for the needs of.'
(https://oxforddictionaries.com>care)

These definitions demonstrate the importance of understanding different attitudes to care and their practical implications.

Whilst you as a carer do want provision for the health and welfare of the older person, this is only part of the process. You need recognition for who you are as a motivator, encourager, emotional supporter and someone who sees the cared-for as an individual. You are trying to create a situation of care and concern, building on a long relationship history which may not always have been positive.

'One of the most difficult challenges was maintaining a tolerable relationship with my mother whilst trying to care for her.'
- Peter -

For the care system, on the other hand, the provision of the services themselves is the focus and the carer is just one contributor. The older person is the central cog, so to speak, of the wheel of services.

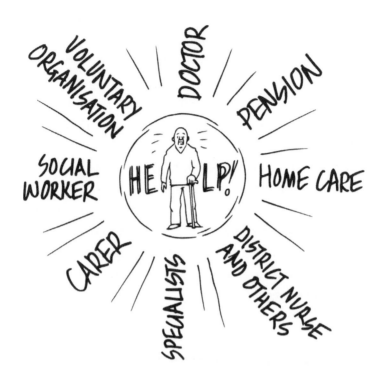

Over the years, this perspective has led to a failed understanding of the importance and needs of carers and lack of communication between the various service providers.

'I walked in and found my usually very positive mother with her head in her hands. She had had four different services calling in that morning. She was exhausted and felt nobody recognised that she was ninety-six years of age. I had to pick up the pieces.'

- Jane -

As a carer you need to have an understanding of the context in which you are operating and your role in it, so as to be able to cope when trying to obtain the care you need for the older person.

Without this understanding, it is possible to end up blaming yourself for not being able to find or use appropriate systems. This feeling of failure can compound the problems which you face.

'Professionals assume you have the knowledge necessary to be a carer. I would have liked help on understanding dementia and even information on how to bathe my mother safely.'
- Nancy -

So you need to recognise that the system in which everyone has to operate is too complicated. It is very difficult to find out who you need to speak to over a specific issue. This is not just mentally and emotionally draining, but physically challenging, as you get tired when being passed from pillar to post.

'Services have become a lot more complicated in the last ten years. I have seen carers lost looking for someone to turn to.'
- Mo, nurse -

Sometimes it is difficult to work out who is responsible for care. Policy makers can assume that there is a network of willing family and community support able to provide care. The practicalities of people's lives today mean that this is not necessarily the reality.

*'When my mother was insistent about returning home
from residential care, despite her complex health needs and
vulnerability, the emphasis of the discussion was on what help I
could and would offer to support her in her own home.'*

- Peter -

It can be difficult for carers to understand where you fit in. You
need to understand that the services are working in a climate
of priority setting and cost cutting that comes from a business
model. Much of care provision today is based around assessment
against specific needs and limited resources. This can appear to
conflict with your perception of the needs in your situation.
Your role may become one of negotiation and coordination.

*'We had four different care companies coming into our home within
a three-year period. There was little consistency of carers and changes
occurred according to the resources the authorities would pay for.'*

- Judy -

SO HOW CAN CARERS NEGOTIATE WITH THE CARE SYSTEM?

- **Know your rights as a carer.**
- **Recognise that there has been a change in approach
  to support and providing care.** If you are to negotiate
  effectively, assertiveness is a necessity, not an option.
- **Look to develop a personal relationship and trust**
  wherever possible between you and the person you care for
  so that you are 'singing from the same hymn sheet', and
  then between you and the professionals/paid workers.

- **Develop your understanding of the role and limitations of the services.**
- **Develop your own personal map of services involved** and how they can be coordinated according to your needs as well as those of the person you are caring for.
- **Identify a key communication point**, particularly someone who is in a position to facilitate coordination.
- **Be clear about the priorities for you as well as the person cared for, and be firm and assertive when negotiating** (or find someone who can do this for you and enjoys this sort of process).
- **Challenge assumptions made about your position as a carer**, know your own boundaries and do not give way to other people's expectations.
- **Enlist all the support you can get** to listen to your frustrations, assure yourself it is not your failings that are causing the havoc and take yourself out for a 'defuse'.

As you think about the scale of the ride, it may seem overwhelming at first. However, getting an understanding of the situation facing you should give you the knowledge to encourage you to step on the rollercoaster with confidence. The following chapters will lead you step by step through the whole experience.

2

. . . .

ENTRY INTO CARING

. . . .

Look before you leap!

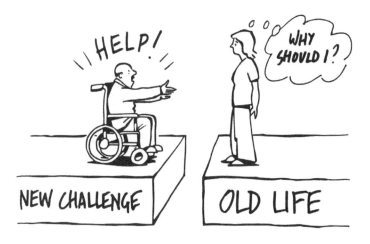

'If I had known what I was getting into, I would never have made such a commitment to the role.'

– Kate –

It can be so difficult when you are suddenly faced with having to recognise that someone who is close to you is getting older and starting to lose their independence. It can be hard to face change of any sort, but when an older person who has previously been capable suddenly needs to be cared for, you can find yourself at a loss, wondering how you can cope and manage this new challenge in your life.

Caring can start with simple practical tasks like help with shopping. The need for support gradually increases over time, until you find caring has taken over your life.

'Mum lived thirty miles away. I didn't drive but would go down on the bus at weekends to help with her shopping initially. As her memory failed and her medication increased, her need for more help and support became crucial. My siblings didn't live locally either and as I didn't work I was expected to take on the central caring role. We tried eventually to have formal carers visit but it was so hit and miss. There was no consistency. I suddenly found myself collapsing under the strain of being a carer.'

- Helen -

Caring can also start as a result of a crisis. It rapidly takes over your life and you have to work out how you are going to handle it.

'I found myself sitting at the kitchen table crying. I was seventy-two with rheumatoid arthritis. I had had a mastectomy, a knee and two hip replacements, and was awaiting a second knee replacement. I now found myself as the main carer for my husband (eighty-two) who had been diagnosed with advanced prostate cancer. I didn't know how I was going to cope.'

- Agnes -

Do you recognise any of the following situations?

- Dad has died suddenly and your frail elderly mother lives alone 300 miles away.
- Your elderly uncle has recently died and your auntie would like you to help her manage her finances.
- An older friend has become isolated and lonely, and needs taking out more.
- You are single, working full-time and live with your elderly parent who has had a serious stroke and is about to return home from hospital.
- Mum has been diagnosed with a chronic condition and you realise that this has long-term implications for her personal independence.
- An elderly relative's physical health is failing and you feel you should help with practical tasks like shopping, cleaning.
- You are elderly and your partner has had a fall and broken their hip.
- Your father's short-term memory loss is becoming a hazard.

If you do recognise any of these, or other similar situations, it is time to consider that you may be joining the ranks of people called 'carers'. This role brings its own constraints, expectations and opportunities. You need to stop and make an honest assessment of your own circumstances. What are the realistic options and constructive choices available to you?

You may be in a partnership, single, have financial constraints, or have other expectations on you. Whatever the circumstances, the role of carer needs to start on a positive note. Whatever your relationship is with the older person, your commitment to care for them should ideally be based on genuine love and care, not obligation, expectations from family, culture, or religion, or drifting into it. Few situations are ideal and some may be very difficult. However, it is possible to prepare yourself for what might be a very long involvement by facing up honestly to the realities of your own personal situation.

'I didn't expect it to last for twenty-six years.'

- Jane -

There are some questions which it would be helpful to ask yourself at this point. It is important from the outset not to do it alone. Seek out close family or friends, or others you can trust to help and support you. This will begin to develop the network you will need and help to ensure that you will not end up isolated.

1. **What is your motivation to care?**
   - Do you think you should, because it is expected of you?
   - Do you want to out of love?
   - Do you have to for practical reasons?
   - Would you enjoy the closer relationship?
   - Do you feel obliged to because you owe it to the older person?
   - Do you want to because it could bring financial gain?
   - Do you need to because you feel guilty?
   - Would you enjoy feeling needed?
   - Do you need to feel needed?
   - Do you already have the skills and cannot ignore the need?
   - Do you feel you cannot do it for any reason?
   - Or for any other reason?

2. **What realistic commitment are you able to make?**
   - What are you physically able to take on?
   - Who else needs you and how?
   - What might you have to give up or put on hold?
   - How will you adapt to the changes in your priorities?
   - How will you maintain your own identity and social contacts?
   - What levels of stress are you currently under?
   - What would be very new and demanding for you?
   - What knowledge/skills do you have or need to develop?

3. **Who else is involved and how?**
   - What if you didn't care? Who would do it? Who would suffer?
   - Are you alone in the role or should sharing with others be agreed from the outset?
   - What are the expectations of all concerned?
   - What is the potential impact of the demands on you of being a carer or on your other relationships?
   - What are others' expectations of you in your role as a carer?
   - How do you feel about the person for whom you are caring?
   - What are the implications of your relationship with them if you become their carer?

4. **What might be the resource implications for you or your family of taking on the caring role?**
   - What are the costs of buying in caring and support services, e.g. home help, gardening, nursing care?
   - How will it affect your working life?

- What financial contributions are available from the person being cared for, yourself, other family members and the benefit system?
- What financial management responsibilities may have to be considered, e.g. power of attorney?
- Are there travel and/or transport implications?
- What housing and accommodation changes need to be considered?

Having answered these questions, you may end up feeling a bit confused and daunted. It can help if your responses are then brought into some kind of action plan. One way of doing this is to do a practical exercise asking the following questions and inserting the answers into headed boxes. This can give you a more organised picture of what is going on and the pressures likely to develop.

So ask yourself the following questions and insert the answers in the blank framework provided at the end of this handbook:

- What are the strengths in my situation that I can bring to the caring role?
- What are the weaknesses which make the challenges of caring more difficult?
- What are the opportunities in the situation?
- What are the threats to my current life?

You can really help yourself see a way forward and make caring easier in the long run, because from the information in the boxes you can begin to make a plan of action taking into account all the factors influencing your situation.

CONSIDER THE FOLLOWING EXAMPLE:

Mary, aged fifty-seven, is married and works part-time. She has three grown-up children living locally, and two grandchildren. Her youngest son, aged twenty-four, lives at home. Mary has three brothers, one who lives a hundred miles away; the other two live abroad. Her father died a year ago. Her mother recently had a fall. She returned home, but has lost confidence, and is starting to struggle with household tasks. Mary's husband Derek helps her with her finances.

STRENGTHS	WEAKNESSES
Good relationship with Mum.	*My brothers are so far away.*
Helpful husband.	*Derek has poor health and is getting*
Mum has good neighbours.	*worse.*
I have a part-time job and love it. It helps	*Mum has limited income coming in.*
our income as well.	*We are somewhat dependent on my wage.*
I have a few good friends.	
OPPORTUNITIES	THREATS
I could seek help from my daughters.	*I may not be able to babysit so often for*
Could my brothers give some financial	*my daughters.*
help?	*I could have to give up my job.*
Neighbours keep an eye on Mum.	*I feel resentful of the changes which caring for*
It's an opportunity to return the care she	*Mum would bring into my life.*
gave me.	*Mum's physical and mental health is*
	deteriorating.
	Mum has lost confidence after her fall.
	How long can Derek go on helping with
	finances when his health is getting worse?

When you have completed the SWOT diagram you start to
have a picture of your full situation. You can then use it to
develop an action plan.

Mary's 'to do' list might look like this:

- Talk to my friend Elsie about how I feel about looking after Mum. I am in danger of being a bit resentful.
- Talk to Mum about her loss of confidence, and see what she thinks she needs. Could an emergency button help?
- Check with Derek about his feelings about looking after Mum's finances, and how he sees my increasing involvement with Mum.
- Discuss with children the implications of reducing child care, and also whether they can offer any support.
- Discuss with boss at work what flexibility I can be given in my hours, and what my employment rights are as a carer.
- Ask my brothers how they can help by keeping in touch with Mum and with me. Maybe they could help pay for a cleaner/gardener?
- Check Mum's neighbours are still happy about keeping an eye on her. Tell them they can always get in touch with me.
- Check with Mum's doctor about her deteriorating health and what she might need.
- Discuss with Mum setting up a power of attorney for finance and health.

Your aim is to set up a system which gives you support, builds on your strengths, and avoids isolation and burn-out. Would you agree with Mary's list? Would you change or add anything? What would your own analysis look like? (Use the blank sheet at the back of the handbook.)

After you have done this and have a to-do list, you may feel a bit overwhelmed. There is a great deal of help out there, so start putting into practice what you will need to learn, and ask for it!

We have put a list of some resources at the end of this handbook, but seek a friend to talk to about your situation, visit your doctor if necessary, go swimming, have a rest, go for a bike ride, or do anything that gives you mental and emotional space.

Caring can often feel like a burden, and may realistically be so at times. However, you need to try to see it as a normal part of life. If you acknowledge the difficulties it may present from the beginning, you can plan realistically the contributions you can make, and where you will need help and support. You may have found the questions about your feelings difficult. Whatever reactions they have triggered will have an effect on the way you handle being a carer. You need to address these at the beginning, otherwise you will only find yourself addressing them later on. Relationships do change, but it is important for all of those involved to see beyond the functional needs and make space for being people together, keeping and developing their own identities. Both carer and cared-for can make their own contributions to the new situation.

'I know I am falling to bits physically, but I am mentally still all here. I am so glad that the family recognise this and come to me for advice. It makes me feel like a wise old bird that still has a role to play.'

- Agnes -

Starting to understand the role of a carer for an older person, and beginning to experience it, is a steep learning curve. You may be feeling more confident and able to proceed. However, as the older person gets increasingly frail, the work becomes more demanding and stressful. It is in the next chapter that we explore ongoing caring, and the range of emotional challenges it can bring.

3

·········

CARING AT HOME

·········

The greatest challenge

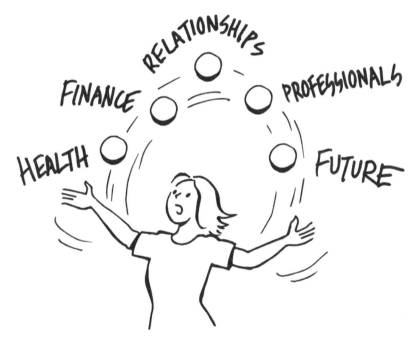

'Although you don't live in the same house, you might as well because you never switch off.'

- Denise -

How does caring reach the parts of you that other experiences do not reach? Once you find yourself in the role of carer, you quickly find that there are no recipes or formats for what you should be doing. Every relationship is unique in what it can offer and in the challenges it presents. The challenge is to keep hold of the vision of what you are doing and why. It is helpful if the carer and the cared-for older person recognise each other's identity and potential contribution. Caring need not be a one-way street. You can try to use each other's strengths to help you get through. This may not always be possible depending on the capacity of the older person being cared for and your relationship with them, but you can try! Quality of life is the key purpose for both you as the carer, and the older person for whom you are caring.

However, you may experience a range of physical and emotional stresses which feel overwhelming.

'As Dad, who had dementia, deteriorated he would become aggressive and hit me. It upset me so much.'

- Lucy -

Identifying these stresses in your own personal situation will enable you:

- to cope with them
- to care effectively and long term if necessary
- to emerge healthily after caring ends.

So what are these demands? They have been identified through a variety of research into carers' experiences. They fall into four main categories which may put a strain on your emotional resources and resilience in different ways. These are:

1. health implications for carers
2. the practical and financial implications
3. the effect on personal relationships
4. relationship with professionals.

1. Health implications of caring

These can have a serious impact on your wellbeing. You may find that you struggle with the physical aspects of the role. Even the carrying of extra shopping, lifting of wheelchairs and domestic chores can take their toll, especially if you are not so young yourself. You may experience feelings of inadequacy as well as tiredness and exhaustion.

'I feel so guilty. Why aren't I glad to be able to give them my time and care, but I'm so tired all the time.'

- Neil -

'At first I really struggled showering my aunt but we tried to make light of it and reduced the feelings of embarrassment felt by both of us by laughing about the fact that I ended up getting as wet as her.'

- Trish -

The Princess Royal Trust for Carers (2001) found that carers sacrifice their own health to maintain the wellbeing of the person they care for. In fact they found that one third of older carers had said that they had cancelled treatment or an operation they needed because of their caring responsibilities. Half of these carers also reported that their own physical health had deteriorated.

'After Dad fell out of bed we got a side guard but he wouldn't have it. It made me so angry because when we found solutions he wouldn't accept them and it put such a physical strain on Mum, especially as Mum had had a minor stroke and had high blood pressure herself.'

- Sarah -

You may experience feelings of disgust when physical accidents occur. This is an emotion which is difficult to admit but is quite common.

'One of my greatest fears was the potential of having to help my mother with personal hygiene tasks. I had no experience or training in how to lift her properly. I was afraid I might hurt her.'

- Natalie -

'After Ben came home from hospital I walked in one day to see Jess with her hands waving in the air shouting look what he has done. Ben was standing there covered in shit and although Jess had took him into the bathroom, with his mind failing he had followed her back through the house, spreading the mess everywhere. I stood there disgusted, thinking I can't clean him up. Then to my relief my husband and son walked through the door and led him back to the bathroom to sort him out.'

- Kate -

Although many carers acknowledge that they get a lot of personal satisfaction from their role, unpaid caring can have a considerable effect on a carer's mental health. The emotional stress can sometimes lead to depression if it goes unaddressed.

For others, giving caring a priority can lead to unfulfilled ambitions and opportunities. Helen felt that giving up work until well into her fifties to care for her mother left her feeling trapped and that life had passed her by.

'By only caring for my mum for years I feel it's too late to start back into any career. My confidence and self-esteem has been battered and I feel left not knowing what I am good at.'

- Rachel -

2. Practical and financial demands

The provision of care for older people raises significant practical and financial issues. The older person is having to adjust to receiving care and having less control in their life. You as the carer may have to involve the family and/or other supporters in exploring the best way forward. Identifying and addressing these issues may reduce emotional stress for everybody concerned. However, it may also increase hidden or previously unexpressed conflict, and you can feel challenged rather than supported.

'In the case of my stepfather, the three older sons wanted me and my husband to undertake all the caring responsibilities. They did not want their father to have help brought in or to go into residential care. They made this very clear that this would affect their inheritance.'

- Bernadette -

'I wanted to do everything to help my mother live at home, but I was not living locally. My brothers were, and they really wanted her to go into residential care because they felt she would be safer,

and they were a bit unsure about taking the responsibility for her care. It was really difficult to come to an agreement and we had to negotiate through the social worker.'

- Annette -

No matter what the circumstances, family relationships or culture, a realistic appraisal of the practical demands needs to be made in order to deal with the situation. For example:

- What happens if your mother starts to lose her sight?
- What happens when your father keeps leaving the cooker on?
- What happens when your partner returns from hospital with a cast on her arm after a fall?
- What happens when your mother starts responding to financial scams on the telephone?
- What happens when your friend cannot drive anymore?
- What happens when your auntie can no longer cope with stairs?

When these kind of issues arise, the first step for everyone involved is accepting that something has to change. This is not easy as it requires letting go of previous lifestyles (almost as hard as Mum deciding she cannot cook Christmas dinner anymore!).

'You are forced to take on tasks you don't like. I hate managing money. My parents had a savings account and their pension. They had never had direct debits. It was a nightmare trying to take on their financial management, especially when they had always been so private about their money.'

- Neil -

Some of the changes you want or have to make may themselves create pressure:

a) Trying to acquire outside help with practical tasks
It can be difficult to find good quality help with trustworthy staff at a reasonable cost. Many older people struggle with modern systems and financial management. Their need for support may stretch your own knowledge and experience.

'It all seems to come down to cost. If you were loaded you wouldn't have to talk to Social Services. Mum just wouldn't spend the money for outside help even though she could afford it; the expectations fell on me.'

- Neil -

Crises can give rise to a number of practical problems which have to be solved in a hurry.

For example, you may come into caring through supporting a parent whose partner has died suddenly, and who needs help with financial management.

'My mum had never even written a cheque and constantly rang me with any bills or phone calls she received concerning these matters.'

- Jane -

In the end Jane accepted help from a cousin and found a financial adviser to help her mother.

b) When additional care is required, financial issues become unavoidable

It is helpful to discuss and plan financial intervention and support as early as possible in order to prevent later problems.

'I found it really helpful to have discussed my mum's financial arrangements and what she wanted immediately after my father died. It was so useful to have things clear from the outset.'

Jane

Whilst the older person may have to think through their financial situation, you as carer may have to face your own challenges:

- You may be using more petrol/transport costs.
- You may be paying for additional equipment and shopping.
- It may be having an effect on your paid work.
- You may have to buy in support for yourself (cleaner, child care etc).

It is important to review these as things change.

'We agreed early on that part of Mum's attendance allowance should be used to pay me for some of the tasks I agreed to undertake.'

- Mary -

A fundamental requirement for ensuring that financial issues do not get beyond control is to ensure that the older person has taken out a power of attorney so that it is clear who has the power to make decisions should they become incapacitated.

When Nancy's mother's mental capacity started to fail, she concluded that she needed to apply for power of attorney. Together they visited a solicitor. Her mother was very confused and the solicitor said her mother was not in a fit mental state and recommended Nancy get an assessment. Nancy paid £250 for a private assessment. She was shocked and upset to discover her mother had mixed dementia. Under the Mental Capacity Act 2005, Nancy successfully applied to the Court of Protection for an order appointing her as deputy for her mother's property and financial affairs at £200 a year cost. She was obliged to prepare a detailed report explaining the decisions made on her mother's behalf on an annual basis and keep accounts and follow the rules for gifts and expenses when acting as deputy. Nancy and her husband found this a nightmare in the first year. Nancy felt that if they had discussed finances with her mother early on, her mother would have been happy to agree to a power of attorney and this could have saved Nancy a great deal of upset and additional work.

3. Implications for personal relationships

Needing to be cared for brings about a change in a person's lifestyle and personal needs. It also brings about a change in relationships, particularly with their carers. There can be a range of emotions and reactions experienced by both of you, which may be difficult to admit.

When the older person begins to fail, whether physically or mentally, they can feel a loss of independence and identity, as well as pain and illness. As a carer you begin to recognise that this deterioration is going to increase. It will apply to more aspects of the older person's life, and require more and deeper levels of care. This may lead to emotional stress for both of you which can impact on your relationship.

'As Mum's health failed, her inability to manage on her own at home increased. Our relationship began to change. After her heart attack she lost her confidence. She made more demands on me to do tasks, some of which she still could have carried out. She would get angry if I tried to encourage her to do things and I would get frustrated and found it emotionally draining constantly trying to boost her confidence and keep her going.'

- Denise -

It may be distressing when you try to continue to do everything to the best of your ability, and the older person appears to have no understanding or appreciation of what you are doing.

'Mum was always concerned to assert her independence, and would say to others that I did very little for her. This led to me exploding in anger, and storming out of the house feeling very guilty. It took a friend saying "oh you have a slice of normal family life" to put the whole thing into perspective for me as a single woman.'

- Jane -

Although Nancy was aware her mother had dementia, she found it very difficult when her mother said cruel things to her.

'I was upset but felt there was always a hint of truth in what she said, and that I had been a disappointment to her.'

- Nancy -

Becoming a carer can result in an increase in your own isolation and in some cases lead to loneliness. The increased demands on your time in the role can affect your own personal relations and friendships. In some cases carers give up paid work to look after the older person and lose even these contacts. You may end up feeling guilty when you take time out from visiting, go out socially without offering to take the older person with you, or even organise respite breaks.

'It got to the stage when I daren't say I was going out for the day with my husband. She made me feel dreadful if we didn't include her.'

- Bernadette -

As the older person's health fails and they become more socially isolated, you may find yourself as their main social outlet – if they have to give up driving, for example, and are dependent on you for transport. The impact of this should not be underestimated. It may limit the opportunities for you to go out socially. However, where there is a positive relationship, a mutual benefit from the need for social activity can be developed.

'When Mum got so that she could not walk very far, I decided to join her in her birdwatching interests, so she could be left with binoculars looking at birds whilst I went off for a short walk, and then we could talk about what we had seen, and share a common interest.'

- Jane -

'My aunt loved a run out in the car. We bought local maps and would wander off occasionally trying out routes we had never been on. Often this resulted in fun experiences on tiny roads or tea at a hidden gem of a café or pub. I learnt so much of the family history on these trips and our relationship benefited from not constantly focusing on domestic chores or hospital appointments. Now looking back it helps to have happy memories to counteract the frustrations and difficulties I did experience when caring for her.'

- Trish -

There can also be wider consequences for a range of relationships with surrounding family, friends and neighbours. If you have siblings, caring for a parent can raise a wide range of issues and affect your interaction. It was common for the people we interviewed that the main caring role fell to one person. Contributions and support from others varied greatly. This can be for a variety of reasons. One sibling may live more locally or is seen to have more time. In some cases a daughter may be expected to do the lion's share of the care.

'Although there was some division of tasks with my sister, my brother did nothing despite the fact that unlike us he had no children and also lived as near to Mum as we did. Mum expected a lot from my sister and I but didn't expect my brother to help in any way. It was so frustrating.'

- Denise -

'My upbringing in a home where I was the only daughter meant that I never questioned that I should remain at home as the carer, giving up my job and marriage prospects.'

- Rachel -

Geography as an influence should not be underestimated. Where families live at a distance, and can only visit at specific times, they may get recognition and a welcome way beyond that normally received by the primary carer.

'My brother and family lived abroad. Their visits were particularly stressful as my mum was intent on everything being perfect for them when they came, played to the gallery while they were visiting, and then collapsed in exhaustion afterwards, leaving me to pick up the pieces. My family then underestimated the stresses of the situation for me and blamed what they saw as my emotional instability.'

- Jane -

Having the main responsibility for an ageing parent may lead to you feeling resentful, particularly where family members discuss their gripes about each other behind each other's back. In such cases it is crucial that roles and boundaries of all involved are set from the outset. Without such consideration, relationships can be damaged long term and it can add stress to an already demanding set of circumstances.

'I was the only one that lived locally and my husband was very helpful. However, the very fact that my brothers appreciated what I was doing and contacted me regularly, allowing me to rant freely about the stresses of the task, helped me no end.'

- Trish -

4. Relationship with professionals

There comes a time when you and your personal support systems have done all you can to enable the older person to live independently in their own home. Their deteriorating health may result in what seems like a revolving door of hospital stays and returning home. A crisis may eventually occur where they end up in hospital for a time, or cannot manage at home with the current level of support. What about you as the main carer? Have you got to the stage where you think, 'I just can't do this anymore'?

It is important to recognise that another period of transition has started, and once again you need to take stock. A reassessment of the situation may conclude that it is time to seek formal paid help. This may not be so easy to do as:

- it entails you acknowledging that you cannot do everything and that you need help
- the person you are caring for may not want strangers in their home and insist they can cope
- both of you may be afraid of change
- other members of the family may object.

Change has to occur to ensure your mental and physical health, and the welfare of the person for whom you are caring. This is inevitably stressful, but can be compounded by the way in which services are delivered in health and social care.

Many of those who work in these services are dedicated and want to provide the best support and care for older people. However, there have been dramatic changes in the provision of health and social care. Resources are limited and services are provided using a business model. It is important to explore and understand the systems through which these services are provided. As a carer you are looking at all the needs of an older person, but a care organisation is there to provide a specific service within legal constraints, e.g. an occupational therapist will look at health and safety around the home, and how to make moving about easier and safer. As more services are involved, whose main focus is on the person being cared for, there is a danger that you can become seen as just another service provider. This can result in a lack of coordination and miscommunication.

'All I seemed to see of the health and care services that were involved in the care of my dad were cuts and incompetence. I learnt to develop a very thick skin dealing with these professionals.'

- Sarah -

'I still feel a real anger towards the hospital. The systems I was trying to work with were awful. I didn't feel supported and there was such poor communication.'

- Hazel -

'One occupational therapist was kind and spared a thought for me. She showed a real insight into the stress I was under, and completed her role effectively, efficiently and with compassion.'

- Peter -

Feedback from carers in research and in our own interviews, has indicated that negotiating a sensible care plan can be very difficult.

'There was no consistency in the carers that came or the times they visited. It was all so hit and miss.'

- Joyce -

When you do obtain help it may be limited.

'I finally got a home help for Mum. When doing the cleaning she wasn't allowed to move furniture and did the minimum in the bathroom. It defeated the object as I had to go and do the difficult and time-consuming jobs myself.'

- Denise -

You can feel very disempowered as a carer. It is easy to forget that the person you are caring for and/or you are actually purchasing these services, and have a right to ensure that they meet the required needs in the way that you would wish.

You can have very positive experiences, however, and where this happens it proves vital to the emotional wellbeing and support of the carer.

'My dad's social worker was a godsend. She saw me as a person, and helped me express and manage my emotions, which helped me cope.'

- Lucy -

Some carers see an improvement in support when the older person comes out of hospital. Several of our interviewees felt that this was because it helped to prevent bed blocking.

'When Mum came out of hospital the crisis team was brilliant. The initial period of returning home was supported by a cost-free package. However, as soon as that period finished it was back to the family to do everything.'

- Martin -

The challenges of caring are varied. Everyone will have different needs for support and resources at this difficult time. In order to cope with the ever-changing circumstances, there is a need to develop personal resilience. This entails looking at what gives you inner strength, what networks of support you have, what practical and financial resources you can draw upon, and what close relationships can be there for you. Where are the gaps in knowledge, relationships and skills and abilities that need to be addressed? The following questions are not exhaustive but by considering them, and maybe implementing just a few of the suggestions, you may be able to relieve some of the pressure on you.

ARE YOU HEALTHY AND LOOKING AFTER YOURSELF?

How can you manage the health implications of your caring role? It is important that you consider both your physical and mental health needs. You cannot always be independent. It is alright to ask for help.

- Do you need a health check?
- Should you seek professional support through your doctor or a counsellor?
- Are there members of the extended family that could provide a listening ear?
- How could friends support you?
- A problem shared can be a problem halved. Is there a local carers' group you could join?
- Are there support systems in your workplace?
- Are you a member of a church or spiritual group where support may be available?
- Can you identify someone who could talk to the older person and encourage them to accept help and recognise your needs as a carer?
- Where are you going to let off steam, and with whom?
- Could you take a little more exercise, even gentle walks, or take up a sport?
- Are there other interests or groups you could join to get a break? You may need not to be so available!
- Could you take regular breaks or book a holiday?
- Is there someone you can really speak honestly with where you can get rid of your frustration?

HOW CAN YOU ADDRESS THE PRACTICAL AND FINANCIAL IMPLICATIONS OF CARING?

There are practical and financial demands on both your life and that of the older person. These frequently lead to high stress levels. It is the arena where it is essential to seek help and support from others.

- Can family, friends, neighbours be encouraged to visit, or take the older person out?
- Can you get help for them to attend appointments and social events?
- Can you get help for either of you with domestic tasks like cleaning or gardening?
- Do you need help with home repairs and maintenance?
- Would food deliveries/help with shopping, ready meal deliveries be helpful?
- What practical equipment would be helpful, e.g. aids around the home for the older person, a lightweight wheelchair?
- Can you divide up any of the above tasks with other family members?
- Can neighbours be involved in any of the above?
- What financial matters need to be considered? What is available?
- What state benefits are available for the person you care for, e.g. Attendance Allowance, or for you, e.g. Carer's Allowance?
- Is the older person able to pay you as a carer if you have to reduce your hours in paid work?
- Can other family members contribute financially to meet care costs?
- Do you need to sort out a power of attorney, a living will, a financial will? This includes you!

HOW CAN BOTH OF YOU MEET THE DEMANDS OF YOUR PERSONAL RELATIONSHIPS?

This is one phase of your life when it is important to stand back and look at how your relationships are being affected. This will enable you to receive support and to develop the emotional resilience to see you through.

- Do you each have your own friendships and are you able to maintain them?
- Where relationships overlap, e.g. with family members, are there issues which need to be addressed?
- Where do you get support for the times when conflict has occurred when the person you care for is feeling the loss of independence?
- How do you maintain and develop the relationship between you, within the changing demands of caring and being cared for?
- Do you have joint interests that you could develop together?
- How do you manage the relationship when you do not get on well, or there are difficulties in communication?

WHAT PROFESSIONAL SERVICES ARE NEEDED TO SUPPORT YOU BOTH?

Involving formal care services can feel extremely daunting and frustrating. The key to it is to get knowledge of how the system works and value your own expertise and experience. Understand that you have a right to challenge and get the specific services required according to the needs of the situation. Do not be afraid of those who seem to be in authority, and develop your assertiveness and negotiating skills. Ask:

- What support is available and/or would you like from the GP surgery?
- Is a formal assessment of the older person's needs through Social Services necessary?
- Would you benefit from a formal carer's assessment for yourself? You are entitled to this.
- Check what benefits you may be entitled to so that services can be bought in.
- Do you need to bring paid carers in as support?
- Explore respite services that may be available.
- Are there local voluntary organisations that may provide support, e.g. sitting services?
- Seek out practical guides or any training on lifting or other physical tasks.
- Are there guides and advice available on chronic conditions and failing mental capacity such as dementia to ensure you are as prepared as possible for future challenges?

Fear of the future can be an unexpected consequence of the demands of caring. What happens when the older person's health fails? What happens if I cannot cope?

'I wasted so much emotional energy thinking about things which might never happen, rather than using my energy to keep things going in the here and now.'
- Mandy -

It is important to look at how things are changing in the situation and your role in it.

'Early on I kept trying to remember the mum I had known all my life and that she had cared for me. I now had the privilege of walking through the final stages of her life with her. This was by no means easy and didn't always work but it did help me.'

- Jane -

It is important that as a carer you look after yourself, otherwise you may not be able to continue carrying out the caring role.

'I was a carer for thirty years and my advice would be "look after yourself whatever it takes. Try and love yourself as much as you can whatever that is for you."'

- Rachel -

Setting healthy personal boundaries and allowing time for personal relationships, family and friends are vital to ensure that your needs and theirs are not neglected. Life will eventually move on from this phase as a carer and it is important that you keep your own life and needs in focus for that future.

Despite all your best efforts, however, there may have been a number of crises, or circumstances with which neither you nor the person you are caring for are able to cope as things stand at home. The difficult necessity of having to consider supported living or residential care becomes the next challenge. It can be a steep climb, which we will deal with in the next chapter.

4

·········

WHEN RESIDENTIAL CARE TAKES OVER

·········

Am I still a carer?

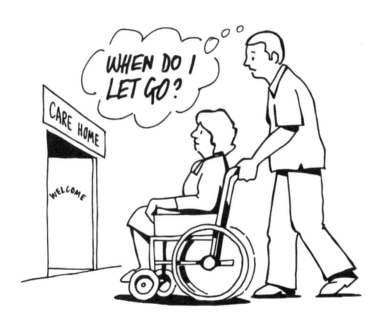

'I felt so guilty when she went into the home. We pretended that she would be going home. She would have been a real risk to herself, so we thought by not telling her that it was a permanent arrangement might help her settle.'

- Jean -

A new stage in the process of caring occurs when it becomes clear that an older person needs more care than can be provided in their home setting. This presents a number of challenges which are not only practical but can create tension in relationships.

Firstly, the time will come for a new assessment to be made which focuses on the needs and energy of you as the carer, as well as the person being cared for.

This ultimately ensures the best care for both of you. It is a really important task, as it makes you think of yourself as a person again. If it is done well at this point it will help later when you are faced with bereavement and loss. Now is the time for you as the carer and, where possible, the person being cared for to take stock. The following questions provide a framework for exploring supported living or residential care in a positive manner.

As a carer you should ask:

- Is the older person at risk and is it possible to monitor the situation sufficiently to keep them safe?
- Have there been any significant changes in your family circumstances?
- Are other relationships at risk as a result of your caring responsibilities?
- Is your own physical or mental health at risk?
- Are your caring responsibilities putting a strain on your finances or affecting your ability to meet family or work commitments?
- Has the all-consuming nature of care made you socially isolated?

Where possible the older person should be helped to consider the need for a move by asking:

- Do they need basic care on a continual basis?
- Do they have significant health needs that residential nursing care would meet?
- Do they need to feel more safe and secure?
- Would they welcome more company and stimulation?

Needing to think about these things may create a situation full of complicated reactions and feelings. This can also bring about a change in family dynamics if the wider family are now involved in the decision-making process. It is useful if others can help. Involving others with some distance from the situation (including social workers where appropriate) may contribute some objectivity.

'Social Services could have done more. We had to constantly chase them. In the end they just gave us a list of homes to contact. Looking at the homes would have been much more problematic if we didn't drive or have the support of family members to come and assess the homes with us. I would recommend people get as much help as possible at this time.'

- Willow -

If the older person is involved in the decision-making process, the decision to move into residential care may be gradual. A range of specific emotions may surface for both the older person and you as carer. Both have to come to terms with the need for change, facing up to the loss of the older person's independence in their own home.

'Mum contacted friends who had gone into residential care and I asked around friends and colleagues who had been involved in sorting out residential care for an older member of their family. This helped us both to ask the right questions and know what we were looking for.'

- Tricia -

If the older person goes into care as a result of a crisis situation, e.g. after a fall and hospitalisation, or does not have the mental capacity to be involved in the decision-making process, much of the responsibility will fall on the main carer with the possible involvement of other family members.

'The home was far from ideal and I felt so bad about that, but with his medical conditions and aggressive behaviour it was the only place that would take him.'

- Neill -

'Guilt overwhelms everything although I knew residential nursing care was the only option.'

- Louise -

Examples like those above highlight the need for shared decision-making, and where possible to share the responsibility and provide support for the main carer at this time of significant change.

Another key feature of this type of crisis entry into care may be the sudden loss of control to the medical profession. Your major task as carer may quickly become more formal, in order to ensure that the older person is seen as an individual. You will want to protect them against institutionalisation, fighting on their behalf to ensure that they are properly cared for.

'My experience of the staff was not very caring and I found myself constantly battling with the home and professionals to care for my friend appropriately and ensure that she kept her identity and was treated like a person.'

- Jane -

Once the decision is made that residential care is the way forward, the second set of challenges occur. Your role and tasks as the carer change rather than disappear.

Finding an appropriate home may be difficult. It is emotionally challenging to undertake a task you hoped you would never have to do. You may have little personal knowledge and limited support depending on where you live. You may be coming to terms with all the emotions about letting go and relinquishing direct responsibility for the older person.

You may have been so busy getting them to think about going into residential care that you failed to recognise your own struggle with feelings of failure yet relief, and guilt for not 'being able to cope'. If you have had no experience of residential homes, then the initial exploratory visits may be shocking.

The following checklist may be helpful:

- Explore the local resources available to you through statutory social services or organisations such as Age UK (see resource list).
- Explore online resources.
- Seek someone to visit with you and offer support – either a social worker or an experienced friend.
- Check out and/or seek someone to sort out the financial implications of going into care with the person cared for.
- Check the Care Quality Commission UK website or their equivalent for their reports on local care homes.
- Explore the possibility of a respite care trial.

Once the older person is taken into a care home and they themselves are learning to adapt, the third set of challenges comes into play.

Physical separation from the person you were caring for whilst trying to maintain your relationship with them introduces new dimensions to your role.

The situation is initially alienating, as much of what you shared is taken away. If you have lived in the same house as the person who has gone into residential accommodation, you can find yourself with an 'empty nest syndrome'. You may be left grieving your life together in your previously shared home. The interdependence of carer and cared-for has apparently come to an end. The loss of control and identity needs to be considered for both of you.

As a carer you may find yourself trying to protect the identity of the cared-for as they enter the residential care environment.

This is emphasised if the entry into care was through a crisis or mental incapacity. Either way, the medical and social care professionals take control, and focus on the older person with the needs. They want to bring their expertise to bear. The carer's knowledge and expertise may be ignored, or distanced. You may experience rejection of all that you have previously done and been, whilst being relieved that you no longer have the responsibility for crisis management.

Because of these changes, defining your caring role when the older person you have cared for goes into residential care is important from the outset. It is important to recognise that whilst the older person has to come to terms with the loss of their home and independence, so too you as a carer will be mourning the loss of your role and many of those things that gave roots and security to everyday life and identity. Recognition of the emotions involved in the situation from both perspectives may assist all those concerned in this period of change.

Your new role and identity can suddenly demand changes to your lifestyle and can present a number of opportunities and sometimes difficulties. Whatever the circumstances it is important to recognise the emotional aspects of dealing with a residential care setting.

Again some key questions may be helpful:

- What practical support does the older person need (like own TV, personal toiletries)?
- How often am I able/should I/do I want to visit?
- How do I ensure that all the appropriate support medical care is made readily available (doctor, optician, chiropodist etc)?
- What new options are available to me for my own life?

- How do I help the older person maintain old relationships and develop new ones?
- How do I build on and develop the good aspects of the home?
- How do I best maintain my own relationships whilst leaving space for the new era to develop?

Eventually the situation will settle down, and you enter the fourth phase of stability (hopefully!).

The person in care has begun to develop a quality of life and new relationships with the staff of the home and other networks.

'Mum went into a care home where the staff cared for her with skill and tenderness despite her persistent reluctance to stay over a period of eight months.'

- Peter -

You now have the beginnings of a normal life back, and some relief of pressure. There are still some challenges, however.

One of the most difficult aspects of the change is that you and the person you care for have entered a world where care becomes a business – 'commodified'. The relationship between the carers/management in the home and the resident can be much more based on a job to be done than on a relationship. Trying to find the balance and negotiate any agreement calmly when such complicated emotions are involved may be very frustrating and emotionally draining.

Financial management can become crucial, both of the older person's affairs and of the contract with the home. It is important to look at who has the right skills and abilities in the new situation. The whole family will need to be involved as the expense affects inheritance.

'There was real conflict in the family. My stepson wanted Dad to stay at home. He had no understanding of the caring required and only visited occasionally. I knew he was concerned about the costs of care and its implications on his inheritance.'

- Agnes -

As the older person gets settled in the home you may have an opportunity to stand back and reflect. If you can, talk through the experience of change with someone. Being listened to can help release tension and any other emotions, including misplaced guilt. If this experience has also triggered other memories, you may need to address these and give yourself permission to do so, taking time to use help if necessary.

'I was so frightened putting my dad in a care home, as I knew my friend still suffered so much guilt because her mother had had such a bad experience in care.'

- Noel -

This process of allowing feelings to surface can help to ensure that you maintain your own identity, and your relationship with the person in care and their carers.

Knowing that your relative is properly looked after can be a relief and a release, and should be treated that way. You have choice about how much to be involved, and an opportunity to rebalance your life. Learning how to do this is really important, as the time will come when the person being cared for will die, and you will be looking at another new phase in your life. The next chapter deals with bereavement, a real challenge on this rollercoaster ride.

5

·········

BEREAVEMENT

·········

The steepest learning curve of all?

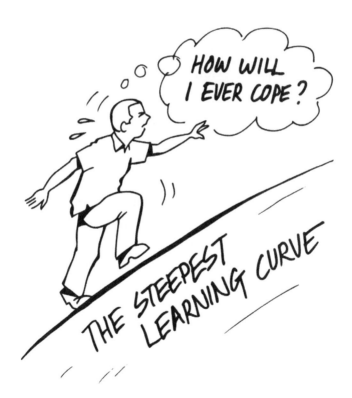

'Cry... holding back the tears can be as exhausting as releasing them. To allow yourself to mourn is essential to your wellbeing and recovery.'

- Shirley Farrier -

Bereavement is a normal experience of life for which we can rarely feel prepared. The immediate demands of the funeral and afterwards leave a lot of practical issues to sort out. Accomplishing these tasks can help you to cope. It is often in the weeks afterwards that intense emotions can emerge, which if left unaddressed and unrecognised may leave you overwhelmed or upset. Friends and family move on, and therefore the opportunities to work through feelings may be limited. As a society we shy away from death and dying. We do not recognise that it is not a single event, but a process, a final passage that can make demands on all our practical and emotional resources for a much longer time than we anticipate. How we cope with it depends on each individual and their circumstances.

Grief and loss are the unavoidable price we pay for love and commitment. The loss of someone with whom we have been intensely involved through the additional carer/cared-for roles can add to the stress in different ways.

Firstly, the intensity and interdependence of the relationship may bring key emotions to the surface. You can suffer a bewildering range of reactions which may include elements of relief, guilt, resentment, anger and sadness. It is important that you give yourself the opportunity to recognise and face these feelings as a helpful way of accepting your loss in your life and dealing with the necessary, if painful, readjustment.

Secondly, the major transition in your role may leave you feeling bereft of more than the person you have lost.

'I have lost my job.'

- Kate -

'Over supper, my brother and I suddenly realised that we were the "elders" in the family now, and did not like it very much!'

- Jane -

Thirdly, you may experience a feeling of being lost as you and others try and reach a new understanding of your identity.

'I am no longer introduced as Mum's daughter, but who and what am I?'

- Sandra -

'Nobody knew how to treat me, now I was not attached to Mum, and I felt so alone and lost.'

- Jane -

Fourthly, relationships with others may have suffered, and resentment, bitterness and different levels of grieving of all those involved can make it difficult to move on.

Fifthly, relationships with organisations which provided, or were supposed to provide, services may have been very stressful.

Anger at their incompetence, lack of communication, poor treatment and so on can entrench you in your own feelings of failure, thus preventing you from moving into healing.

'My siblings gave me very little support in caring for our father, but were very evident at the funeral and the reading of the will.'

- Rita -

'Now Mum has died, my sisters and I want to make a formal complaint to the hospital. However, my siblings are expecting me to do all this, and that's causing resentment.'

- Roisin -

Working through all these, as well as our personal sorrow and loss, is often more than we can or should do on our own. There are some key principles, however, which can help:

1. Accentuate the positive
Identify, write down and be thankful for the good experiences and aspects of relationships that you had with the person you were caring for, the people around you both and the services. This helps to prevent the negative issues dominating, and allows you to grieve healthily with thankfulness. You may find expressing this through letter, email, diary, creativity of some kind, a helpful release.

2. Identify difficult relationship issues which have occurred
Identify the difficult issues that have occurred in relationships. Face up to how you may have contributed to them, and be prepared to say sorry if necessary. Identify the circumstances where anger and bitterness arise/arose. As you are able, forgive those who have hurt you, or the person you cared for. You may need a good listener alongside you to help you with this.

3. Reflect on your experience of the services you received
Experience of poor services in the last stages of your loved one's life can be devastating, as can behaviour during the aftermath – organising the funeral and so on. The early stages of bereavement may be the first time that you have been able

to recognise all that went on, and feel the anger and injustice. Again, it can be helpful to write down specific instances and work through what could help you feel better. You will need to recognise the pressures on the people concerned as well as on yourself, and distinguish between what is the effect of wider policy and what is downright bad practice by an individual. Then you may be able to forgive both the individuals and/or the organisations/system.

You may wish to make a formal complaint eventually, with help from others.

Dealing with all these at once may be overwhelming. A simple awareness of the stages of bereavement can help you as a former carer to understand what you are going through and help you work through the process bit by bit.

'I had a kind of mental washing line on which I hung each issue I was grieving about. As I dealt with each one, I folded it up and put it in the basket. It was great when I had an empty line!'
- Sandra -

Each stage is characterised by particular emotions. If you recognise which of these are significant for you, it can give you more confidence to work through them and see a way forward.

1. Immediately after bereavement

The experience can be one of shock and numbness.

'The final stage happened so quickly I was left in a state of disbelief and numbness which I felt for a long time.'
- Helen -

This may be compounded by the fact that as the carer, you may need to deal with funeral arrangements, wills, house clearance and so on. You find yourself doing this on automatic pilot, putting your own grief on hold. A lack of recognition and support at this early stage of the process can have long-lasting effects on how a bereaved carer can move on.

'Mum just died in the hospital bed and I walked out of the cubicle where I was handed a leaflet on bereavement. No one spoke to me so I walked out of the hospital. It wasn't until I reached the bus stop that I broke down and the tears flowed.'

- Helen -

Sometimes it is very difficult to face the reality that the person has gone.

'You've lived in the caring role for so long your mindset seems to carry on even when they have died. I remember taking her clothes for burial to the undertakers and I said "I've put in a vest to go under her blouse, please use it as she always feels the cold". I must have sounded so daft.'

Trish

Shirley Farrier, a hospice social worker in *A Time to Grieve*, highlights the experience of some bereaved people she has supported. She identifies in them a sense of apathy, leaving them feeling listless and flat as the reality of the death emerges more clearly. She suggests that this can be positive as a sign of beginning to adjust. She recommends that showing emotion is important.

Feelings of relief immediately after a bereavement can be very common but feel very wrong. After the demands of caring and watching over someone as they fail, it is natural to feel relieved when they are out of their struggle, and you no longer have the demands on you which may well have become more than you felt you could handle.

'Even now three years on I don't think I have grieved. My caring role went on for so long and took so much out of me I am still coming to terms with not having this all-consuming role that I feel nothing but relief.'

- Bernadette -

You can also experience a sense of searching for what is lost, and wanting to continue the normal pattern of life, for example, like unconsciously continuing to set an additional place setting at the dinner table. This acute and powerful emotion of yearning for the person who has gone can be exhausting.

'I would be sitting in the garden, and would hear the tapping of Mum's walking stick coming down the drive, and my peace and new freedom would be interrupted.'

- Sandra -

2. Working through the pain

Regret characterises many aspects of our lives, whether it is sadness about opportunities missed, or feelings that you could have done something better. Caring for an older person is no different. The role of carer is an extremely demanding one. Carers are not trained professionals and yet have to learn so much and deal with so many competing demands. It would be impossible to do every aspect of the role perfectly, but it is hard to recognise this when you are still very close to the situation.

'Here I am at seventy. I cared for Mum since my dad died when I was nineteen. I have felt "what is there to live for?" I missed my chance to marry and I would have loved to have a family. I wish I had had the confidence to stand up and set boundaries for my own life and needs.'

- Rachel -

'I should have fought for better care for her in the hospital.'

- Hazel -

Regret for what was left unsaid or undone is common to carers.

'I didn't do enough, but thinking that makes me sad because I know I did everything I could.'

- Judy -

Linked with regret can be a sense of sadness not only that the person has gone from your life but also for what you feel you have not done.

'It has left a sadness that the day she died I popped in at home before going to visit her in the home and she died without me being there.'

- Nancy -

Sometimes the parting process is multi-layered, and can trigger feelings from previous bereavements.

'I had been a carer for my aunt for twenty-three years. In her last illness she was taken into hospital and I spent a great deal of time with her. She insisted I go away for a night to a friend's

party. When I returned she was unconscious. We moved her to a hospice and I stayed with her constantly day and night for seven days. On the last morning I joked we would become permanent staff or they might throw us out for being there so long. I then said I was popping to the loo as the nurses came in to make her comfortable. As I was returning the nurses called for me. I rushed into the room but she was gone. I felt cheated that at both stages I hadn't had the opportunity to say goodbye. The same had happened to me with the death of both my mother and father. The nurse tried to comfort me saying it was quite common for patients to seem to wait and pass on in this way. Even now although I feel that I have moved on, I will always have regrets about this.'

- Trish -

Anger is also a common response to grief. It may be triggered by a number of things.

You may be feeling angry towards the person who has died, because it feels as if they have abandoned you.

Many can experience feeling angry with family members.

'My brothers only wanted to be involved after the caring was over. They were only interested in dealing with the money.'

- Carrie -

You can feel angry towards yourself as the carer.

'I should have kept her out of hospital.'

- Jane -

This may be accompanied by a sense of failure. Carers are often quick to focus on having let their loved one down. They forget that they are not a trained expert yet have fulfilled their role admirably to the best of their ability.

'I feel angry that I never had space to think and possibly try and do things differently.'

- Martha -

In contrast the anger may be towards the services or lack of support received from formal caring agencies.

'I had to spend a lot of time forgiving consultants and nurses for not giving her the right medication and endangering her life, which meant I was forever in a battle when I was in need of support.'

- Jane -

Guilt is perhaps the most painful companion of bereavement. Even in the most positive relationships between an elderly person and their carer, this emotion can surface during the grieving process.

'Guilt overwhelms everything. I have a real fear of losing control.'

- Pat -

'Even now the guilt is sometimes overwhelming. I know I'm not yet at the stage to feel better about any of it.'

- Doreen -

'I was not there when Mum died. Yet I did so much. It's hard to feel this horrible feeling of guilt.'

- Nancy -

'Now some time has passed. I see I was unwell at the time and was struggling with other work and family commitments. I did what I could. It is time to let the guilt go. It is not achieving anything, only eating me up and stopping me from moving on with my life.'

- Mary -

Resentment does not always die with a bereavement, and can get in the way of moving on.

'I feel she has stolen my best years. Life passed me by when I put my mother first. Now having never married or developed any career I weep thinking it is now too late.'

- Rachel -

'All our lives Dad controlled and bullied us. We tried to be good carers to the end but I still hold the regret that we missed out. Family life could have been so much more if our relationships had been better.'

- Sarah -

Feeling isolated can also be a feature of bereavement.

'Early on, the practical steps of arranging the funeral and taking care of the estate keep you focused and busy. You are surrounded by other people giving you company and support. Afterwards it can be a different matter.'

- Mary -

Isolation may be particularly difficult if you are an older person who has cared for a partner.

'I can't bear being in the house on my own. I just have to get out.'

- Agnes -

You may suffer great loneliness, deprived not only of your dearest companion but also many of your generation. Daughters and sons may have lost contact with other members of the family, and may not be able to be honest about what they feel.

3. Beginning to accept your loss

If you begin to have a sense that the fog is starting to clear, and that there may be life ahead, you are beginning to come to terms with and accept your loss. This phase is characterised by a sense of relief. You are not using all your energy controlling your emotion, and putting a face to the world.

'When I could shop in the supermarket opposite the hospital without going round like a zombie, I felt that I was moving on.'

- Sandra -

A sense of release may also characterise your acceptance, because you can be glad that the person you cared for is out of their pain, and you can work on your own agenda.

'At last I have my wife back and we can now put each other first.'

- Martin -

When you have faced up to your key emotions, you are able to 'change the record'. You stop telling yourself and others about all the negative experiences, and you are able to let them go and put them in the past.

'I felt a real resentment to the step relatives who were never there for the caring, but were immediately there for the will. It does not bother me anymore. I see their lost opportunities.'

- Tina -

You may have a sense of moving into a new identity. People do not see you as a carer anymore, and neither do you. You can feel that you have some energy to redirect into new things.

'I've had a lot of time to stand back and reflect. I did what I could. Now I need to think about me, find myself, maybe take up something creative.'

- Helen -

You may tentatively accept that a new phase of your life has started and that you can move on. The person you cared for is no longer your primary concern when you wake up. You know you can make plans for the day and feel the glimmerings of hope.

HOW DO WE LET GO?

Understanding the process of grieving is all very well, but how can we work through it and move on? You may have identified with some of the feelings expressed above, and may have others of your own. If you work through the grid at the end of the chapter, it should help you to feel that you have some control of the process.

It is normal to feel a range of emotions to varying degrees after the death of the person for whom you have cared. They should be regarded as steps along the way of bereavement to a healthy new phase of your life. There are some general principles, however, which can help:

- Be patient with yourself.
- Take time to rest and sleep.
- Look after your health as a reminder that you are of value.
- Think of ways to help you remember the person you have lost. Dedicate a bench somewhere nice where you can sit and reflect. Plant a tree in their memory. Try and express your feelings in a tangible creative way – a photograph album, or a journal.
- Avoid immediate major changes to your life for the first year if possible.
- Avoid looking for or being given others to care for to replace the role you have lost.
- Don't feel pressure to 'get over it'. Take time, as long as YOU need.
- Don't allow anyone to tell you how to feel, and don't tell yourself how to feel either.

- Find a listener with whom you can share your feelings without shock or embarrassment, preferably someone who has had experience of the caring role.
- Ask for help when you need it (carers have to unlearn the habit of being the 'fixer').
- Plan ahead for triggers that may make you feel sad. Birthdays, holidays.
- Try and remember what you used to enjoy, or think of things you might want to try, and, starting small, have a go.
- Remember it can all take longer than you think or want, but it is your restoration that matters.

At any stage, you may feel that things are not going as you would like and you need extra help. You may experience any of the following:

- Desire to withdraw from other people
- Low mood, depression or suicidal thoughts
- Loss of appetite or excessive eating or drinking
- Continued sense of exhaustion and tiredness
- Disturbed sleep patterns
- Keeping over busy
- Lack of concentration
- Tearfulness
- Inability to acknowledge your loss

DO NOT STRUGGLE ON REGARDLESS. SEEK HELP FROM SOMEWHERE/
SOMEONE YOU TRUST (SEE RESOURCE LIST).

In caring for an older person at the final stage of life we can learn so much: respect for one another, and the courage and the capacity to accept, endure and to love. You could even suggest that in many ways we can learn from people who are ill, how to help, and from people facing death, how to live. It can be an opportunity for development and growth for all those involved. We need to be mindful, however, that we are often taught to suppress our emotions. The pain of grief needs to find a channel and not be avoided but faced and shared. It is so much healthier in the long run.

It is important to get to the point of feeling able to let go and move on, which we will explore in the next chapter.

WORKING THROUGH THE STAGES OF GRIEF

If you look at the grids below and identify those relevant to you, add others, then use the other two columns to identify situations which are triggering the feelings, and what you might do about them. This may help you to see where you are in the process and give you a sense of control over it. This is the first step in ceasing to be overwhelmed by your loss. Remember there is no right place to be. Each of us is different in how long it takes, and how we face it. We have to be kind to ourselves!

STAGE 1: INITIAL GRIEF

FEATURES OF STAGE	ISSUES IDENTIFIED	ACTION TO TAKE
Shock and numbness		
Loss/searching		
Yearning		
Denial		
Apathy/ listlessness/fatigue		
Anger		
Relief		
Other		

STAGE 2: WORKING ON THE PAIN

FEATURES OF STAGE	ISSUES IDENTIFIED	ACTION TO TAKE
Regret		
Contentment		
Sadness		
Guilt		
Resentment		
Failure		
Isolation		

STAGE 3: LEARNING TO ACCEPT

FEATURES OF STAGE	ISSUES IDENTIFIED	ACTION TO TAKE
Relief		
Release		
Faced up to key emotions		
Sense of new identity		
Acceptance of a new phase in life		
Other		

6

· · · · · · · · ·

MOVING ON

· · · · · · · · ·

Now it's over, where do I go from here?

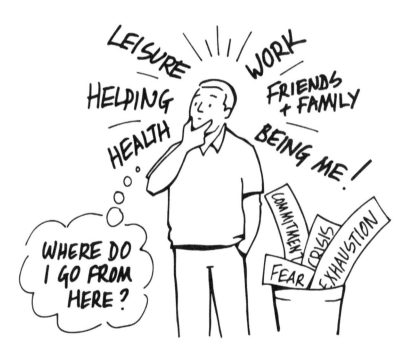

'Grief is part of love and love evolves.
Even acceptance is not final, it continually shifts and changes.'

- Megan Devine -

Moving on from your role as a carer is extremely challenging. The priority now has to be you and your needs. You can start thinking about yourself for the first time in years, and this may feel very strange and disorienting. The key is to actively tackle this change rather than drift into it. Easier said than done!

There is clearly no correct way or timescale prescribed for grieving and moving on, and the process is unique for each person. However, being aware of the wide range of emotions that others experience may help you recognise your own issues and understand that they are common for many carers going through this process.

Each person is unique and much will depend therefore on aspects such as:

- the length of time you were a carer
- the experiences and effects on relationships during this time
- the changes that caring brought about in your lifestyle
- experience of the support services.

1. The length of time as a carer
There is a big difference between a short sharp emergency period of caring and a long-term complex experience, sometimes leading from caring for one person into caring for another.

'I still can't grieve for Mum because Dad is in a home with dementia and keeps asking where she is.'

- Neil -

'Because I was a carer for so long, it has surprised me that it has taken me four years to feel that I can start to move on.'

- Trish -

2. The experiences and effects on relationships during this time

These can have a very significant impact. Where a relationship was very interdependent, the gap left by bereavement can be overwhelming.

'Because my life totally revolved around my mother, I found myself very isolated after her death, but I am finding that good friendships, going to church and other activities are helping me to move forward.'

- Rachel -

Sometimes people who are being cared for have negative reactions which can have a big impact on a carer.

'Caring for my mother has really knocked my confidence, and I don't know what I am good at anymore.'

- Helen -

'It is now two and a half years since my mother's death. I still feel tearful whenever I think about her and guilty for not meeting her needs as she saw them, as we never had a very good relationship.'

- Peter -

3. Changes that caring brought about in your lifestyle

Becoming a carer often means you have to change the structure to your life. It can be quite disorienting when you face changing your lifestyle again.

'I've lost my job. Who am I now?'

- Kate -

'I still cannot go out for the day in the country on my own.'

- Jane -

'Since I lost my dad I have lost my income and my home, have been declared fit for work and I have no idea where to look for a job.'

-Michael -

4. Experience of the support services

The battles with hospital, care and community systems during caring can leave us with a load of anger, frustration and distress which can make it difficult to move on.

'Several years on, I still experience waves of anger at the way my parents were treated by the hospital and the care system. I need to let it go.'

- Lucy -

'I still get upset not just at the poor practice of all the services involved with my mother, but at the lack of their compassion when she died. I still feel emotional stress from this.'

- Peter -

'I was treated with such care and compassion immediately after the death of my aunt by the hospice staff that it lifted any feeling of guilt I might have had that I was not there the moment she died.'

- Trish -

5. So where do you start when you want to move on?
The first step in dealing with these issues is for you to reflect and to revisit your relationship with the person you cared for. This will help to ensure that you lay a healthy foundation for your new life ahead.

So ask yourself:

What was the relationship?

How dependent were you on that person in your life?

Have you accepted the reality that the person has gone?

Are you still in a period of feeling the pain of grief or loss?

Are you adjusting to an environment without the person who has died?

Are you withdrawing your emotional energy from the person who has died and now thinking of new horizons?

(Adapted from Worden 1991)

Having responded to these questions you will have a better idea how you feel about the person who you cared for and their absence. How do you feel about yourself and your own needs? You may have forgotten how to identify these, or even see them as worthwhile. Now is the time to recognise that the next stage is all about you.

'As my friend said to me, my new mantra must be "me! me! me!"'

- Denise -

It is helpful to reflect on which rituals and routines may trigger feelings of grief and loss so that you can be prepared. It may be the obvious occasions like birthdays and anniversaries, or times of celebration. It may be the unexpected, like going back into the house after a good time out, or seeing a favourite film on the television. It may be just normality like the downtime after nine o'clock at night, or even a mealtime routine.

'My friend was really helpful. She said "ring me in the downtime" because she knew what it was like living on her own.'

- Karen -

Being a carer may have had a significant effect on your surrounding relationships. What needs to be addressed so that it does not block you moving on? Do you need to clear the ground with relatives or friends where relationships have slipped because of the pressures? Are there past relationships you could reactivate, or new ones you need to seek out? You may not feel very confident, but all you can do is try!

The caring process may have left you feeling empty and exhausted. In order to move on you will need to re-energise, and this means being kind to yourself, remembering what gives you an emotional, physical or spiritual lift, and ensuring that you make time and space for the process.

'I knew I was moving on when I started to be able to play the piano again.'

- Jane -

It could be useful to revisit your SWOT analysis, but this time with you at the centre.

Ask the following questions:

- What are the strengths which will help you to move on?
- What are the weaknesses which might hinder you moving on?
- What are the opportunities available to you now?
- What are the threats to developing a way forward?

An example might look as follows:

Geraldine is fifty-two. She was the primary carer for her mother, for ten years. In the last twelve months her mother has died and her husband has retired. Her daughter has married and is expecting her first child and her son has gone to university. She finds herself in an empty nest with time on her hands. Physically she has a bad back from lifting her mother. Her husband's pension is not substantial, so they need to find extra income for the household. She also feels quite isolated, as she had very little time for a social life when the children were at home and she was a full-time carer.

STRENGTHS	WEAKNESSES
My children no longer a full-time responsibility.	*I have been out of paid employment for eight years.*
I have learnt a lot from looking after Mum and feel ready to move on.	*I have a bad back and feel very tired.*
I find it difficult to see what strengths I have although Freda says I am really good with people.	*I have lost my confidence. I realise that I have been grieving for my mum all tangled up with the kids leaving home. I guess I need to face up to this somehow.*
OPPORTUNITIES	THREATS
I think I should look for a course or something, so I could get my confidence back.	*My daughter wants to go back to work full-time after having the baby, and she seems to want me to be full-time carer. I am not sure I should do this.*
My husband and I have time to be together, and maybe do something new together.	*We have reduced income.*
I think I really will enjoy being a grandparent.	*My husband is still adjusting to retirement, and he is under my feet.*

How would you advise Geraldine?

For us, her to-do list might look like this:

1. I have to get a check-up at the doctor re my back and the tiredness.
2. I am feeling a bit lost, and I need to talk to someone outside the family, about how I feel overall. Maybe Freda will help. She likes meals out as well, which would help me get out and about again.

3. My husband and I could do with sitting down and talking about our plans for the future both financial and social. We both need some space to develop into our new life together, and possibly time apart to develop our own interests.

4. I need to talk with my daughter about looking after my grandchild and set some boundaries about how much I will do. I don't have to feel guilty!

5. I am terrified, but sometime I need to explore courses/part-time work. I need to remind myself what I used to like doing, and think about what I would like to try.

6. Most of all I need to remember I am free to be me and start behaving like I believe it.

How then can you move on constructively? A framework can help the planning process.

If you work through the following four interrelated elements you may be able to identify each small step that can lead to moving into a new phase of your life.

1. **How do you feel about yourself now?**
   - Has caring left you with a sense of failure, or are you conscious of new skills learnt and a job well done?
   - How can you build on the positive, and address the issues that have affected your confidence?
   - Where did/do you get your sense of self-esteem from other than being a carer? Personal interests? Employment? Friendships? Family? Just being you?
   - Have you forgotten where you ever got it from, and feel utterly lost?
   - Be assured, you do not need to be alone in the process, as there are many avenues to explore (see resource list).

2. What sort of support do you think you need now?

- Have you any health issues which you have neglected during caring or which have emerged since?
- Do you have existing friends who have been with you throughout and you want to be with you in the next stage?
- Do you want new friends who will not be part of your history, but just see you as you?
- Would you like to seek out a support group for people who have had similar experiences in bereavement, loss and trying to move on?
- Would you benefit from personal counselling?
- Would a new activity/social group be helpful?
- Could you reignite your spiritual life and/or seek support from a church?

3. What will you do with all the space in your life?

When you were caring, you will have experienced huge pressure to respond to everyone else's needs immediately. The end of that role brings a void and space which can be frightening. The danger is that you or others feel the need to fill the empty space which the caring role has left. Now is the opportunity to give yourself time to recuperate and revalue yourself. It is about finding space for the development of the new directions which your life is going to take. The way of taking space will vary hugely. It may be shutting yourself in the bathroom in a warm bath, taking a country walk, meditation, listening to music, or just doing nothing at all. Doing it in your own time and not allowing others to dictate the pace or direction is crucial. The purpose is for you to make conscious decisions about your way forward, rather than falling into whatever comes along.

'On reflection, I think I would have benefited from having two days away from everybody and everything, just to get my head straight.'
- Annette -

4. How do you develop your new identity?

When you are a carer, your identity becomes enmeshed in that of the person you care for.

'When I was introduced it was always as my auntie's niece, not by my first name.'
- Trish -

As you move on, one of the challenges is to see yourself, and for others to see you, as an individual, separate from the caring role.

If you have kept your relationships and activities going during caring, you will have a foundation to build on. If the pressures have meant that you have been isolated, you need to give yourself permission to refind your identity and explore who you want to be now. This will need to include the people around you, who may make the assumption that you are now free, and therefore are capable of moving on. They may need prompting that you need some support and/or companionship on the way.

5. How do I know that I am moving on?

A new phase of your life is ahead of you. This can be terrifying, empowering, or even exhausting just thinking about it. However, you owe it to yourself to move forward in the most positive way possible. You have been in practical mode for so long that you may want to leave your feelings behind, because it is so hard to face them. In order to move on, however, now is the time to stop, breathe and reflect, taking as much time as you need to find YOUR way forward. It is so hard to put yourself first and to do what is best for you and not just what is expected of you. Draw on your skills, energy and experience from your caring. You have much to offer YOURSELF. This is the final stage of your rollercoaster ride. There may be ups and downs but being nice to yourself may result in you finishing the journey hopefully with a smile. It takes time, but every small step counts.

7

· · · · · · · · ·

LEARNING FOR CARE

· · · · · · · · ·

We are all in it together

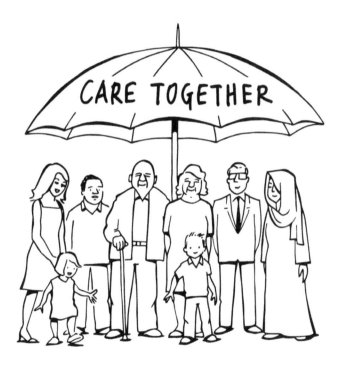

'I was really encouraged by my mother's doctor who put the emphasis on her quality of life and not just on specific health needs.'

- Jane -

Writing this book has meant that we have been immersed in the individual experience of many carers, including ourselves. Whilst we have wanted to offer support to those still involved, the issues arising have been so similar, that we have felt it necessary to look at how our society can create a better context for care.

Care of the elderly has become a topical issue because extended life expectancy has resulted in a change in the age balance in society. At the same time, there is a pressure on health and community resources, families and housing. Caring for older people is going to become increasingly a normal experience of life. In order for this not to be seen as a burden, preparation for caring and being cared for has to be an integral part of our lifelong learning. This has to be not just about the tasks that have to be fulfilled, and the related service delivery, but about the recognition of the relationships that are necessary between everyone involved.

It is important to be able to contribute what you can and receive what you need, wherever you are in the care system (whether informal or paid carer, or someone who provides services). All sections of society need to recognise this concept of reciprocal care whether physical, emotional, or intellectual.

There are several issues which need to be addressed if we are to create a fulfilling and positive context for care.

1. Learning for care needs to start very early on in our lives and be integrated into every stage

The dynamics of family life has changed. In many cases, families are more dispersed, and generations are therefore not as familiar with each other. There has been increased reliance on the state to provide care. The reduction of state provision of residential care for the elderly and increased emphasis on community care means that there is a need for society to re-engage with the idea of the family caring for each other from the cradle to the grave.

Ageing is currently expressed in negative terms as being a financial and social burden on society. Whilst there is a reality in this, the related stigma ensures that we do not see ageing as a natural process. In the later stages of life we deserve to be seen as a contributing individual who now needs additional support.

'When my aunt was in the hospice, I ensured that there was a photograph of her in her early days as a pharmacist and another of her large extended family to remind people who she was and not just this dying aged body in a bed.'

- Trish -

In order to change attitudes and create effective care, we need to promote opportunities for good relationships between the generations at every stage of life.

2. The concept of quality of life has to be reviewed

The danger in society today is that we value people for how active they can be, not for who they are. Older people are driven into hyperactivity in order to conform to the image of youthful vigour. As long as you are healthy and active, you are valued, rather than recognising the range of contributions all can make.

We need to look beyond age and ailments and see the person and their potential. Every age has needs for care and a contribution to make.

> *'At Busy Bees Nursery in Chichester the children do all the usual things like reading, drawing and playing. But three times a week they toddle off to a nearby care home to spend time with the residents. The partnership is proving a great success for the children and the elderly people.'*
> (*BBC Breakfast*, 29 November 2017)

3. We need a concept of care which is relational and reciprocal rather than transactional and based on service delivery

The most important thing about care is people. The danger of concentrating on cost and efficiency has led to the over strain and frustration which are so common for everyone involved. Care works best when it is based on the relationships between people.

To do this effectively, real time has to be factored in to enable people to listen to one another, provide appropriate support and deal with emotions as well as the tasks.

The difficulties of trying to implement a more relational approach to care cannot be over-estimated. If we want to create an environment where the focus can be on mutual recognition and relevant and efficient help and support, we need to readdress the following:

1. Consistency in services

One factor that many of the carers we interviewed raised was lack of consistency in services, whether it was seeing the same GP at their local surgery or having the same carers visit them in their homes. This prevented the development of good communication and understanding of specific care needs, reduced efficiency, and added stress for workers and carers alike.

'There was no consistency in the carers provided for my mother, and in the end we cancelled them.'

- Hazel -

Where services are planned with an understanding of the importance of relationships in the care process, there can be a more effective use of resources, and a more supportive environment for carers and the staff involved.

2. Boundaries

In a growing environment of fear of litigation, the need for extensive legislation and the danger of abuse allegations, the focus on boundaries is crucial. Agencies have set very clear defensive boundaries on what they can and cannot do. However, a balance must be sought which is based on mutual trust and relationships. Otherwise it can potentially lead to boundaries that focus on the task and the problem to be solved, not including the feelings and needs of the person being cared for.

'My aunt would go to a lovely nursing home in the Lake District for respite. I walked in to collect her and the first thing she said was "Can I have a hug?".'

- Trish -

'We are becoming professionals that are hidden behind our work roles with everything subsumed under tasks rather than building trust and relationships.'

- Moira -

How can we avoid becoming technical people hidden behind barriers and role definition, everything subsumed under tasks rather than trust and relationships?

3. Time constraints

Even for carers where there is a personal connection and relationship, the struggle to focus on the feelings and social needs of the person for whom they are caring can become difficult. Having work, family and other commitments means that carers can end up rushing around dealing with the practical tasks and losing person-to-person interaction.

'I would rush in with shopping, sort the laundry, make her tea, with little time to just sit and chat knowing that she must feel lonely sometimes living on her own with little mobility.'

- Bernadette -

Similarly, professional carers have competing demands and limited time, which makes it difficult to consider anything other than the immediate problem to be addressed.

'You can't do the job properly, the way you used to do it.'

- Mo, nurse -

We have to recognise that for effective service you cannot avoid the importance of listening and hearing and that this takes time.

4. Coordination

Those who have contributed to this book highlighted the lack of coordination between services and the difficulties that this caused for carers and their families as well as professionals.

> *'There was no joined-up writing in the many services who were involved with my father. I had to keep repeating myself to each professional because they did not share any information.'*
>
> **- Sarah -**

As people struggled to find their way through the system it was increasingly difficult to develop a constructive and supportive relationship which improved the care.

There needs to be a review of how services are organised and managed so that everyone can work together.

5. Support available

We all learn defensive behaviour when we do not have appropriate support. This can have a serious effect on working together in care. Carers need a safe place to voice when they feel that they do not know what they are doing. They need to be confident in the people who are offering support and it needs to be easily available.

The focus for carers in the professions, on the other hand, is on managerial assessment and appraisal. How do you carry the load? There is the need to build opportunities for mentoring, counselling. There needs to be an opportunity for workers to share and offload the emotions from what are very emotional situations.

6. Resource limitations

Whilst recognising the realities of the current climate, it is being acknowledged that asking people to work in the challenging context of care only on a cost-benefit analysis based on task and function is neither efficient nor effective.

'It was clear that the carers were frustrated because they kept apologising for the little time they had to do the tasks and hated not having the space just to talk to us.'

Joyce

The rising evidence of stress at work, health problems of voluntary carers and recruitment problems calls for an urgent review of care from a different perspective in order not to waste money and people's lives.

Facing these issues feels overwhelming for us all, and there are major challenges ahead.

However, we can start by reflecting on what is good practice. A starting point could be the following framework, 'The Four As'.

ATTEND	ACKNOWLEDGE
Be focused *on the individuals and not distracted (e.g. by phones, paperwork).* **Listen** *attentively and patiently. Do not interrupt, despite their communication difficulties, lack of confidence.* **Think** *about how your response might make someone feel before you say it.*	**Respond** *to the initial apparently minor problem in order to build trust.* **Recognise** *the feelings behind the anxiety being expressed.* **Demonstrate** *that you have heard what they have said and are feeling.*
AFFIRM	**APPRECIATE**
Identify and recognise *the individual's personality, experience and knowledge.* **Reassure** *them of their capacity to cope with the situation.* **Treat people as capable adults** *and be mindful of the dangers of patronising them.*	**Seek to understand** *why they behave as they do.* **Provide positive constructive feedback,** *using standards everyone understands.* **Do not judge or condemn,** *but look for the positives.*

If you are involved in caring for someone, some people are like gold dust:

- Friends who are willing to listen to the frustration and hurt and pain without judging.
- Family who are willing to do little things – DIY, gardening, visiting, bringing a meal.
- Friends or family who continue to see the elderly person as a whole person with whom they still love to interact.
- Nurses, doctors, paid carers who listen, hear real needs, recognise the person, encourage and sustain.
- People who are being cared for who listen, respond, encourage helpers and retain a sense of humour.
- Carers who remain open to help, share and walk with all those involved.

There is general agreement that the social care system is under extreme pressure, and more of that strain is falling back onto carers.

> 'Around one in eight adults is a full- or part-time carer, often juggling work and family too, and saving the economy over £132 billion a year.'
> (Dr Melanie Jones, *Woman's Weekly*, 17 June 2018)

It is important to recognise that we will all fail to be all that we should or want to be. We will need resilience, encouragement, patience, and the willingness to change and adapt. We can only ensure that carers and those who work with them emerge healthily if we create a positive environment of valuing one another.

In the current climate, it is easy to be critical, broken, bitter, and to blame and concentrate on failure. We can, however, choose to learn from and support one another and through building on the positive in small ways, begin to create change.

Useful UK Resource List

Age UK
www.ageuk.org.uk
0800 022 3444
A national voluntary organisation which provides a wide range of information and services for older people.

Alzheimer's Society
www.alzheimers.org.uk
0300 222 1122
A care and research charity for people with dementia and their carers.

Caring for older relatives
www.nhs.uk/live-well/
Practical guidance and support.

Carers Direct
Helpline 0300 123 1053
A helpline for carers about social care and support.

Carers' Trust
https://carers.org
Access to quality support and services to carers.

Citizens Advice Bureau
www.citizensadvice.org.uk
0344 477 2020

A network of 316 charities across the UK to provide free confidential information and advice to assist people with money, legal, consumer and other problems.

College of Occupational Therapists
www.cot.co.uk
0207 357 6480
Helps find an occupational therapist and advises on home adaptations/equipment.

Cruse Bereavement Care
www.cruse.org.uk
0844 477 9400
Emotional support and information for bereaved people.

Dementia UK
www.dementiauk.org
0207 697 4160
Provides specialist advice and support on dementia.

Department for Work and Pensions Bereavement Service
www.gov.uk/browse/benefits and www.gov.uk/power-of-attorney
0345 606 0265
Carries out eligibility checks on surviving relatives for benefits and help with funeral costs.

Discover a Hobby
www.discoverahobby.com
A site with 220 ideas for a new interest.

Disability Living Foundation
www.dlf.org.uk
0300 999 0004
Advice on equipment.

Healthtalk
www.healthtalk.org
The impact of being a carer; topics include caring for someone with a terminal illness, dying and bereavement.

Macmillan Cancer Support
www.macmillan.org.uk
0808 808 0000
Aims to help everyone with cancer live life as fully as they can. Provides a range of services, including a support line, nurses, online community and financial support.

Marie Curie
www.mariecurie.org.uk
A charity which provides support and care to people with terminal illnesses and their families.

Mind
www.mind.org.uk
Help for mental health problems. What challenges do carers face in helping someone else?

NHS Choices
www.nhs.uk
Your health and choices.

National Hospice and Palliative Care Organisation

www.nhpco.org

Hospice services (care/respite and support for the terminally ill and their families).

Samaritans

www.samaritans.org

Tel 116 123

Confidential non-judgmental support for people in distress twenty-four hours a day.

Silverline

0800 470 8090

Confidential free helpline for people over the age of fifty-five, twenty-four hours a day, seven days a week.

Turn2us

www.turn2us.org.uk

0808 802 2000

Help to access benefits, grants and other help.

The Relatives and Residents Association

www.relres.org

0207 359 8136

Supports care home residents and their relatives.

References

British Broadcasting Corporation (2017) Busybees Nursery Partnership, Chichester. *Breakfast News* (viewed 29 November 2017).

Care definitions [online] http://oxforddictionaries.com>care (accessed 3 April 2017).

Devine, M. (2014) 'Have you heard you are not alone in grief? It isn't really true.' [online] www.huffpost.com.>entry>death (accessed 12 November 2014).

Jones, Dr M. (2018) 'How to Care for Carers', *Woman's Weekly* (issue 17 June 2018).

Princess Royal Trust for Carers (2001) Carers Trust – Caring about older carers – Providing support for people caring in later life. [online] http://professionals.carers.org>sites>files (accessed 4 May 2019).

Worden (1991) 'Psychological theories of grief', K260 *Death and Dying*, Book 1 The Social Context of Death and Dying. Open University 2009.

Bibliography

Cohn-Sherbok, D. and L. (2007) *What Do You Do When Your Parents Live Forever?* O Books, John Hunt Publishing Ltd.

Cooke, L. (2009) *Bereavement – The Essential Guide*, Need to Know Publications, Forward Press Ltd.

Farrier, S. (2005) 'Is it alright to listen to me as well?' The United Reform Church, London.

Highe, J. (2007) *Now Where Did I Put My Glasses? Caring for Your Parents – A Practical and Emotional Lifeline.* Simon & Schuster UK Ltd

Hunt, J. (2013) *Grief: Living at Peace with Loss.* Rose Publishing/ Aspire Press.

Jacobs, B. J. (2006) *The Emotional Survival Guide for Caregivers: Looking After Yourself and Your Family While Helping an Aging Parent.* The Guildford Press.

James, W.J. and Friedman, R. (1998) *The Grief Recovery Handbook: The Action Program for Moving Beyond Death, Divorce, and Other Losses including Health, Career, and Faith.* Harper Perennial.

Kubler-Ross, E. and Kessler, D. (2005) *On Grief and Grieving.* Simon & Schuster UK Ltd.

Long, W. (2015) *A Gift for Carers*. Austin Macauley Publishers Ltd.

MacKinlay, E. (2012) *Palliative Care, Ageing and Spirituality: A Guide for Older People, Carers and Families*. Jessica Kingsley Publications.

Marriott, H. (2003) *The Selfish Pig's Guide to Caring: How to cope with the emotional and practical aspects of caring for someone*. Piatkus.

Pavy Claibourne, C. (2016) *Purses and Shoes for Sale*. Acadian House Publishing, Louisiana.

Smith.H and Smith.M.K (2008) *The Art of Helping Others*. Jessica Kingsley Publications.

Whitman, L. (ed.) (2010) *Telling Tales about Dementia: Experiences of Caring*. Jessica Kingsley Publications.